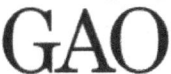

I0425842

June 2012

VA/DOD FEDERAL HEALTH CARE CENTER

Costly Information Technology Delays Continue and Evaluation Plan Lacking

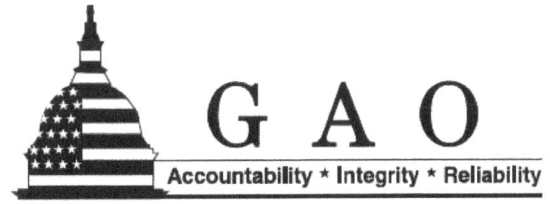

GAO-12-669

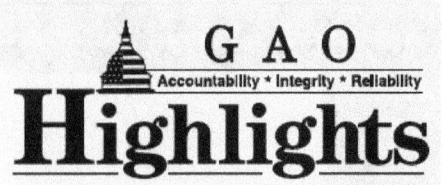

GAO
Accountability * Integrity * Reliability

Highlights

Highlights of GAO-12-669, a report to congressional committees

VA/DOD FEDERAL HEALTH CARE CENTER

Costly Information Technology Delays Continue and Evaluation Plan Lacking

Why GAO Did This Study

The NDAA for Fiscal Year 2010 authorized VA and DOD to establish a 5-year demonstration to integrate VA and DOD medical care into a first-of-its-kind FHCC in North Chicago, Illinois. Expectations for the FHCC are outlined in the Executive Agreement signed by VA and DOD in April 2010.

The NDAA for Fiscal Year 2010, as amended by the NDAA for Fiscal Year 2012, directed GAO to report on the FHCC demonstration in 2011, 2012, and 2015. This is the second of the three reports and examines (1) to what extent VA and DOD have continued to implement the Executive Agreement to establish and operate the FHCC and (2) what plan, if any, VA and DOD have to assess the provision of care and operations of the FHCC.

To conduct its work, GAO reviewed FHCC documents; interviewed VA, DOD, and FHCC officials; and reviewed related GAO work.

What GAO Recommends

GAO recommends that VA and DOD (1) determine the costs associated with the workarounds required because of delays in implementing IT capabilities laid out in the FHCC Executive Agreement; (2) develop plans with clear definitions, specifications, deliverables, and time frames for IT capabilities required by the Executive Agreement but not yet defined; (3) develop and agree to an evaluation plan, to include all performance measures and standards to be used in evaluating the FHCC demonstration; and (4) establish measures related to the cost-effectiveness of the FHCC as part of their evaluation. VA and DOD generally concurred and noted steps to address GAO's recommendations.

View GAO-12-669. For more information, contact Debra A. Draper at (202) 512-7114 or draperd@gao.gov.

What GAO Found

Officials at the Department of Veterans Affairs (VA) and Department of Defense (DOD) Captain James A. Lovell Federal Health Care Center (FHCC) have continued to make progress implementing provisions of the Executive Agreement's 12 integration areas, but delays in the information technology (IT) area have proven costly. Specifically, for 6 integration areas, all provisions have been implemented. Some of these areas were implemented at the time of GAO's 2011 report, including establishing the facility's governance structure and patient priority system, while 2 areas—quality assurance and contingency planning—were more recently implemented. In addition, 5 integration areas, such as property and fiscal authority, remain in progress. However, as previously reported by GAO, there have been delays implementing 1 of the integration areas—IT—which have resulted in additional costs for the FHCC, although the FHCC has been unable to quantify the total costs resulting from these delays. Despite an investment of more than $122 million for IT capabilities at the FHCC, VA and DOD have not completed work on all components required by the Executive Agreement, which were to have been in place in time for the FHCC's opening in October 2010. These delays have resulted in additional costs and administrative burden for the FHCC because of the need for workarounds to address them. There also are other IT capabilities required by the Executive Agreement that are ill-defined and for which plans have not been established.

Although they are required by the National Defense Authorization Act (NDAA) for Fiscal Year 2010 to assess the FHCC at the end of the 5-year demonstration, VA and DOD officials said the departments have not yet established an evaluation plan. Officials told GAO that in addition to the performance data already being collected from 15 integration benchmarks established by the Executive Agreement, the departments also expect to consider other factors; however, these factors, which may include performance measures, have not yet been established. VA and DOD officials also have not yet established the standards, such as target scores for the benchmarks, the departments will use to evaluate FHCC performance. GAO has previously found that well-defined measures and standards are essential to a sound evaluation plan. Furthermore, without VA and DOD agreement on the measures and standards, FHCC leadership is unable to track progress and make any midcourse adjustments to improve performance in areas VA and DOD have determined are necessary for the FHCC's success. Although including measures of FHCC costs in the evaluation would be consistent with the FHCC's purpose, VA and DOD departmental priorities, and federal financial accounting standards, no such cost measures have been established for evaluating the FHCC.

_____ **United States Government Accountability Office**

Contents

Figures

Abbreviations

DOD	Department of Defense
FHCC	Federal Health Care Center
HEC	Health Executive Council
IT	information technology
JEC	Joint Executive Council
MTF	military treatment facility
NCVAMC	North Chicago Veterans Affairs Medical Center
NDAA	National Defense Authorization Act
NHCGL	Naval Health Clinic Great Lakes
VA	Department of Veterans Affairs

June 26, 2012

Congressional Committees

The Departments of Veterans Affairs (VA) and Defense (DOD) expanded their efforts to share health care resources in 2010 following congressional authorization of a 5-year demonstration to more fully integrate VA and DOD facilities located in proximity to one another in the North Chicago, Illinois, area. As authorized by the National Defense Authorization Act (NDAA) for Fiscal Year 2010 (NDAA 2010), VA and DOD facilities in and around North Chicago were integrated into a first-of-its-kind system known as the Captain James A. Lovell Federal Health Care Center (FHCC). Although DOD and VA have shared resources at some level since the 1980s,[1] the FHCC is unique in that it is the first fully integrated federal health care center for use by both VA and DOD beneficiaries,[2] with an integrated workforce, a joint funding source, and a single line of governance. In addition to delivering integrated health care services to both VA and DOD beneficiaries, this unprecedented partnership is expected to offer lessons for decision makers about whether this is a model of care that might be effective if replicated at other VA and DOD locations. Among other things, the NDAA 2010 requires the Secretaries of VA and Defense to submit a report to the House and Senate Committees on Armed Services and Veterans' Affairs by October 2015, the year in which the demonstration ends, to include an assessment of the demonstration and a recommendation as to whether the FHCC should continue.[3]

VA and DOD signed an Executive Agreement in April 2010 that outlined the FHCC's structure. Beginning October 1, 2010, the new structure integrated services previously provided by the former North Chicago VA

---

[1]The Veterans' Administration and Department of Defense Health Resources Sharing and Emergency Operations Act was enacted in 1982. See 38 U.S.C. § 8111. The Department of Veterans Affairs was previously known as the Veterans Administration.

[2]VA beneficiaries include veterans of military service and certain dependents and survivors; DOD beneficiaries include active duty servicemembers and their dependents, medically eligible National Guard and Reserve servicemembers and their dependents, and military retirees and their dependents and survivors. Active duty personnel include Reserve component members on active duty for at least 30 days.

[3]See Pub. L. No. 111-84, § 1701(d), 123 Stat. 2190, 2568 (2009).

Medical Center (NCVAMC) and its community-based outpatient clinics and the Naval Health Clinic Great Lakes (NHCGL) and its associated clinics, as well as services provided by a new ambulatory care center constructed by DOD.[4] The FHCC reported providing care to more than 86,000 patients in its first year of operation (October 2010 through September 2011), including about 25,000 veterans and 59,000 DOD beneficiaries, including Navy recruits.[5]

NDAA 2010, as amended by the NDAA for Fiscal Year 2012 (NDAA 2012), requires that we review and assess the progress made in implementing the Executive Agreement and the effects of the agreement on the provision of care and operation of the facility, and issue reports based on those assessments in 2011, 2012, and 2015.[6] We first reported in July 2011[7] on the status of the FHCC's integration efforts and found that for the 12 integration areas defined in the Executive Agreement,[8] 4 had been implemented, 7 were in progress, and 1—information technology (IT) integration—was delayed. We also found weaknesses in the tool created to collect and report performance results and recommended that the FHCC reexamine its process for assessing and reporting performance to ensure accurate and meaningful information. In addition, we recommended that DOD seek a legislative change to designate the FHCC as a military treatment facility (MTF) to eliminate the need for burdensome workarounds to address several administrative

---

[4]The NHCGL includes a main clinic and three branch clinics that provide health care services to Navy recruits, as well as active duty personnel and their families.

[5]In addition to veterans and DOD beneficiaries, the FHCC reported providing care to approximately 2,000 other patients, including FHCC employees.

[6]NDAA 2010—Pub. L. No. 111-84, § 1701(e), 123 Stat. 2190, 2568 (2009)—required GAO to report annually beginning in 2011; NDAA 2012—Pub. L. No. 112-81, § 1098, 125 Stat. 1298, 1609 (2011)—amended that reporting requirement to include reports in 2011, 2012, and 2015.

[7]GAO, *VA and DOD Health Care: First Federal Health Care Center Established, but Implementation Concerns Need to Be Addressed*, GAO-11-570 (Washington, D.C.: July 19, 2011).

[8]The 12 integration areas are (1) governance structure, (2) access to health care at the FHCC, (3) research, (4) contracting, (5) quality assurance, (6) integration benchmarks, (7) property (i.e., construction and physical plant management), (8) reporting requirements, (9) workforce management and personnel, (10) contingency planning, (11) fiscal authority, and (12) information technology.

challenges that arose because the FHCC lacked such a designation.[9] Specifically, we reported that the FHCC encountered challenges in the areas of managing beneficiary co-payments, contracting to meet temporary staffing needs, using drug pricing arrangements, and clarifying providers' authority to sign medical readiness forms for active duty Navy servicemembers.

In this second required report, we address the following questions:

1. To what extent have VA and DOD continued to implement the Executive Agreement to establish and operate the FHCC?

2. What plan, if any, do VA and DOD have to assess the provision of care and operations of the FHCC?

To determine the extent to which VA and DOD have continued to make progress in establishing and operating the FHCC, we examined the 12 integration areas (and the provisions within each area) outlined in the Executive Agreement and assessed the FHCC's progress in meeting them. Specifically, we reviewed VA and DOD policies pertaining to FHCC operations; meeting minutes documenting discussions of FHCC, VA, and DOD officials about patient care and operations; and financial planning documents, such as the operating plan and budget.[10] For the areas we noted in our prior report as having been implemented, we reexamined these for any changes that might affect their current status. We also reviewed our earlier work, including our first report on implementation progress, and a separate 2011 report specifically examining IT capabilities and planning for the FHCC integration.[11] In addition, we interviewed officials at VA, DOD, and the FHCC about continued progress in establishing and operating the FHCC.

---

[9]According to DOD policy, an MTF is a medical facility, owned and operated by DOD, established for the purpose of furnishing medical care, dental care, or both to eligible individuals.

[10]In the area of financial systems, we did not perform a financial audit of the FHCC, but rather assessed its progress in establishing and operating a model for joint funding.

[11]See GAO-11-570, and GAO, *Electronic Health Records: DOD and VA Should Remove Barriers and Improve Efforts to Meet Their Common System Needs*, GAO-11-265 (Washington, D.C.: Feb. 2, 2011).

To determine what plan, if any, VA and DOD have to assess the provision of care and operations of the FHCC, we interviewed officials at the FHCC, VA, and DOD regarding the provision of care and operations, standards used to measure and assess performance, and plans to evaluate and report results. We also reviewed relevant documents that describe the plans for measuring the FHCC's performance in delivering care to patients and for assessing the operations in support of care delivery. In addition, we examined best practices for program evaluation, mainly within federal agencies, including some specific to demonstrations.[12]

We conducted this performance audit from November 2011 to June 2012 in accordance with generally accepted government auditing standards. Those standards require that we plan and perform the audit to obtain sufficient, appropriate evidence to provide a reasonable basis for our findings and conclusions based on our audit objectives. We believe that the evidence obtained provides a reasonable basis for our findings and conclusions based on our audit objectives.

Background

VA and DOD have a long-standing history of sharing health care resources to provide services to their beneficiaries. However, the FHCC is unique among VA and DOD collaborations to deliver health care services in several ways, notably its level of integration, the way it is funded, and its governance structure. The Executive Agreement, signed by the Secretaries of both departments, contains provisions to be met in 12 integration areas regarding specific aspects of FHCC operations, including establishing a governance structure and combining VA and DOD staff into a single, joint workforce. The FHCC's leadership remains directly accountable to VA and DOD individually, through formal reporting relationships, and jointly, through oversight and advisory entities comprising VA and DOD officials.

---

[12]GAO, *Limitations in DOD's Evaluation Plan for EEO Complaint Pilot Program Hinder Determination of Pilot Results*, GAO-08-387R (Washington, D.C.: Feb. 22, 2008), and *Tax Administration: IRS Needs to Strengthen Its Approach for Evaluating the SRFMI Data-Sharing Pilot Program*, GAO-09-45 (Washington, D.C.: Nov. 7, 2008).

FHCC Established a New Level of Sharing for VA and DOD	VA and DOD have been authorized since the 1980s to enter into sharing agreements with each other to improve access to, and the quality and cost-effectiveness of, health care provided by the two departments. Since that time, VA and DOD have entered into a number of sharing agreements to provide services—such as emergency, specialty, inpatient, and outpatient care—to VA and DOD beneficiaries and to reimburse one another for the cost of such services. Starting in the 1990s, VA and DOD expanded their sharing efforts to include "joint ventures"—locations where sharing agreements are in place that encompass multiple health care services for VA and DOD beneficiaries. The FHCC is one of 10 joint venture locations across the country.[13]

The October 2010 launch of the FHCC demonstration established a new level of sharing and integration for VA and DOD. Specifically, the FHCC is unique among other VA and DOD joint ventures in three key ways:

1. The FHCC's integration of the provision of care and operations represents the highest level of collaboration among the 10 VA and DOD joint ventures. For example, the FHCC has a more integrated staffing structure than any other joint venture site.

2. The FHCC has a joint funding source, to which VA and DOD contribute, unlike the other joint venture sites, which each have separate VA and DOD funding sources. NDAA 2010 established the Joint DOD-VA Medical Facility Demonstration Fund (Joint Fund) as the funding mechanism for the FHCC, with VA and DOD both making transfers to the Joint Fund from their respective appropriations.[14]

3. The FHCC operates under a single line of governance to manage medical and dental care, and has an integrated workforce of approximately 3,100 civilian and active duty military employees from

---

[13]The other nine joint venture locations are Anchorage, Alaska; Fairfield, California; Key West, Florida; Honolulu, Hawaii; Las Vegas, Nevada; Albuquerque, New Mexico; Biloxi, Mississippi; Charleston, South Carolina; and El Paso, Texas. Charleston became the newest joint venture when it was added in 2011.

[14]The Consolidated Appropriations Act, 2012 provided funds for VA and DOD to transfer to the Joint Fund for fiscal year 2012. Pub. L. No. 112-74, div. A, § 8104, div. H, §§ 224, 225, 125 Stat. 786, 830-31, 1158 (2011). Prior to the enactment of the Department of Defense and Full-Year Continuing Appropriations Act, 2011, the FHCC received funding from VA and DOD through an alternative funding mechanism outlined in the Executive Agreement.

both VA and DOD.[15] None of the other joint venture sites have integrated governance structures; rather, they maintain separate VA and DOD lines of authority.

Executive Agreement

In April 2010, the Secretaries of VA and Defense signed the Executive Agreement that established the FHCC and defined the relationship between VA and DOD for operating the new, integrated facility, in accordance with NDAA 2010. The Executive Agreement contained provisions in 12 integration areas regarding specific aspects of FHCC operations (see table 1).

Table 1: Key Provisions of Federal Health Care Center (FHCC) Executive Agreement Integration Areas

Integration area	Key provisions
Governance structure	FHCC leadership structure and advisory bodies
Access to health care at the FHCC	Patient priority system and eligibility of members of the uniformed services for care
Research	Institutional Review Board approval and policy for the protection of human subjects
Contracting	Departments of Veterans Affairs (VA) and Defense (DOD) responsibility for contracting support
Quality assurance	Accreditation and oversight from external entities and credentialing and privileging of health care providers
Contingency planning	Emergency and disaster management and security
Integration benchmarks	Completion of 15 integration benchmarks may occur before 2015
Property	Construction, transfer of property, and physical plant management
Reporting requirements	VA and DOD reports to congressional committees and Comptroller General reviews
Workforce management and personnel	Staffing, training, and the transfer of DOD civilian personnel to VA
Fiscal authority	Budgeting, joint funding authority, and reconciliation
Information technology (IT)	Administrative and clinical IT, including efforts to achieve interoperability between VA and DOD systems

Source: GAO.

Each of the 12 integration areas contains a number of specific provisions describing how the FHCC should be jointly operated by VA and DOD. Some provisions have designated deadlines, while others do not. For example, within the IT integration area, the Executive Agreement included provisions identifying three specific IT capabilities that VA and DOD were

---

[15]This 3,100-employee figure is an FHCC estimate including civilian employees, active duty servicemembers, and contractors.

to have in place by opening day of the FHCC, October 1, 2010 (for example, medical single sign-on, which would allow staff to use one screen to access both the VA and DOD electronic health record systems) while other provisions (such as those for financial management and outpatient appointment enhancement solutions) had no scheduled due dates.

FHCC Oversight

As established in the Executive Agreement, the FHCC's leadership and workforce remain directly accountable to both VA and DOD (see fig. 1). The FHCC Director, a VA executive, is accountable to VA for the fulfillment of the FHCC mission, while the Deputy Director and Commanding Officer, a Navy Captain, is accountable to DOD. In addition, the Joint Executive Council (JEC) and the Health Executive Council (HEC) provide oversight for all of the joint ventures, including the FHCC. The JEC is made up of senior VA and DOD officials and provides broad strategic direction for collaboration and resource sharing between the two departments. The HEC, a sub-council of the JEC, provides oversight for the specific cooperative efforts of each department's health care organizations—VA's Veterans Health Administration and DOD's Military Health System. The HEC has organized itself into a number of work groups to carry out its work and focus on specific high-priority areas of national interest.

Figure 1: Federal Health Care Center (FHCC) Oversight Structure

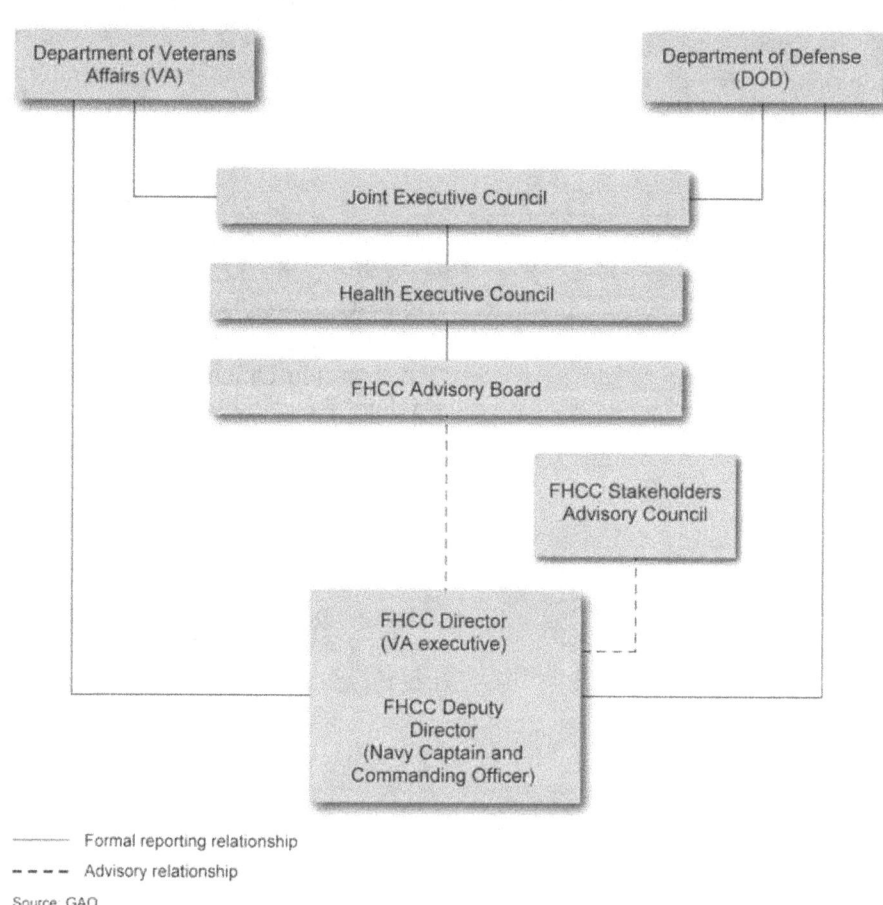

Formal reporting relationship
Advisory relationship

Source: GAO

Notes: Since our 2011 report, the FHCC Advisory Board has become a working group of the Health Executive Council, formalizing its reporting relationship. Some oversight of the FHCC within VA is conducted by Veterans Integrated Service Network 12 and within DOD by the U.S. Navy Bureau of Medicine and Surgery.

The FHCC Advisory Board, a HEC workgroup co-chaired by and comprising senior officials from VA and DOD, was created specifically to provide guidance and support to FHCC leaders and to resolve issues that arise at the FHCC. The Advisory Board provides guidance for the integration and operations of the facility, including monitoring the FHCC's performance and advising on issues related to strategic direction, mission, vision, and policy. It also serves as a communication link between the FHCC and VA and DOD executive leadership by reporting on FHCC activities to the HEC. FHCC issues that are not able to be

GAO-12-669 VA and DOD Federal Health Care Center Update

resolved by the Advisory Board are elevated to the HEC for final resolution. The Stakeholders Advisory Council also provides feedback on how well the FHCC is meeting customers' needs and VA and DOD missions. The Stakeholders Advisory Council is made up of members from various regional and local organizations representing FHCC interests, including representation from local government, TRICARE, and two nearby VA medical facilities.

Further Progress Has Been Made Implementing the Executive Agreement, but Costly IT Delays and Lack of MTF Designation Continue to Pose Challenges

Eleven of 12 integration areas are now either "implemented" or "in progress." The remaining integration area, IT, remains "delayed," as it was at our last review, resulting in costly and time-consuming workarounds. DOD's decision not to seek an MTF designation for the FHCC, as we had recommended in our July 2011 report, has resulted in continued implementation challenges.[16]

All but 1 of the 12 Executive Agreement Integration Areas Are Implemented or In Progress

FHCC officials have implemented or made progress implementing 11 of the 12 Executive Agreement integration areas. Specifically, FHCC officials have implemented 6 integration areas, meaning all associated provisions in the Executive Agreement have been met. Five of the integration areas are in progress, meaning some, but not all, associated provisions have been met, with FHCC officials maintaining or making additional progress meeting the provisions in each integration area. The 1 integration area not implemented or in progress is IT, which is delayed, meaning at least one provision had a deadline provided in the Executive Agreement that was not met. This integration area is discussed in more detail later in this report. (See fig. 2.)

---

[16]See GAO-11-570.

Figure 2: Status of Federal Health Care Center (FHCC) Implementation of Provisions for the 12 Executive Agreement Integration Areas, as of May 2012

Integration area	Implemented	In progress	Delayed
Governance structure	X		
Access to health care at the FHCC	X		
Research	X		
Contracting	X		
Quality assurance	X[a]	X	
Contingency planning	X[a]	X	
Integration benchmarks		X	
Property		X	
Reporting requirements		X	
Workforce management and personnel		X	
Fiscal authority		X	
Information technology			X

Source: GAO analysis.

Note: Integration areas that are categorized as "implemented" are areas in which all the identified provisions in the Executive Agreement have been completed, those categorized as "in progress" are areas in which at least one provision has not been completed, and those categorized as "delayed" are areas in which at least one provision had not met a deadline provided in the Executive Agreement.

[a]In our prior review conducted in 2011, the status of this integration area was "in progress."

Six Integration Areas Are Implemented

FHCC officials have implemented all provisions in 6 of the 12 Executive Agreement integration areas. Of these 6, 4 were integration areas we previously reported as implemented: (1) governance structure, (2) access to health care at the FHCC, (3) research, and (4) contracting. The two other implemented integration areas, quality assurance and contingency planning, moved from in progress at the time of our last review to implemented in this review. Integration areas we previously reported as implemented have remained in that status by maintaining activities or policies that meet the associated provisions in the Executive Agreement.

For example, in the area of governance structure, the Stakeholders Advisory Council meets quarterly as required by the Executive Agreement and in another integration area, research, existing policies remain in place. Since our 2011 report, the FHCC met two additional required provisions for the quality assurance integration area: (1) officials obtained accreditation for the integrated facility by relevant external accrediting bodies—the Commission on Accreditation of Rehabilitation Facilities, and The Joint Commission[17]—and (2) FHCC officials reviewed the FHCC's policy on professional practices.[18] In addition, FHCC officials have established a formal agreement to outline the jurisdiction of VA and DOD related to the security program for the FHCC campus, as the Executive Agreement requires. (See table 2.)

---

[17]The Commission on Accreditation of Rehabilitation Facilities and The Joint Commission are independent organizations that accredit health care organizations and programs.

[18]The FHCC is required by the Executive Agreement to review its policy on professional practices, which deals with staff certification and training, 1 year after the FHCC became operational to determine if it meets the Navy and FHCC mission requirements.

Table 2: Federal Health Care Center (FHCC) Executive Agreement—Status of Key Provisions of Currently Implemented Integration Areas

Integration area	Status of key provisions as of July 2011[a]	Status of key provisions as of May 2012
Governance structure[b]	FHCC leadership structure and advisory bodies were in place.	Maintained establishment of leadership structure; continued to meet provision for the Stakeholders Advisory Council to meet at least quarterly.
Access to health care at the FHCC[b]	Patient priority system to ensure access was in place and FHCC maintained its "pipeline to the fleet" readiness goal by monitoring the medical readiness of enlisted Navy recruits.	Continued to meet provisions related to patient priority system and the "pipeline to the fleet" readiness goal.
Research[b]	Institutional Review Board approval and policy for the protection of human subjects were in place.	Continued the existing policies related to the Institutional Review Board.
Contracting[b]	Department of Veterans Affairs (VA) responsibility for contracting support established.	Maintained implementation of contracting provisions, with VA continuing to oversee contracting support. The Department of Defense (DOD) is responsible for personal services contracts.
Quality assurance[c]	Accreditation and oversight from external entities were ongoing and policies on credentialing and privileging of health care providers were in place.	Met final two provisions: (1) accreditation as a joint facility by relevant external accrediting bodies—the Commission on Accreditation of Rehabilitation Facilities and The Joint Commission—and (2) review of the FHCC's policy on professional practices.[d]
Contingency planning[c]	Emergency management personnel, training standards, and programs were in place. Officials were working on a formal agreement outlining the jurisdiction of VA and DOD related to FHCC campus security.	Met final provision: formal agreement outlining the jurisdiction of VA and DOD related to FHCC campus security established.

Source: GAO.

[a]See GAO, *VA and DOD Health Care: First Federal Health Care Center Established, but Implementation Concerns Need to Be Addressed*, GAO-11-570 (Washington, D.C.: July 19, 2011).

[b]We reported this integration area as implemented in July 2011 (see GAO-11-570).

[c]We reported this integration area as in progress in July 2011 (see GAO-11-570).

[d]The Commission on Accreditation of Rehabilitation Facilities and The Joint Commission are independent organizations that accredit health care organizations and programs.

Five Integration Areas Remain In Progress

Five other integration areas in the Executive Agreement remain in progress: (1) integration benchmarks, (2) property, (3) reporting requirements, (4) workforce management and personnel, and (5) fiscal authority. Each of these integration areas was also in progress at the time of our first report in July of 2011. FHCC officials have actively maintained past progress while continuing to work toward implementation of the provisions in the Executive Agreement associated with these integration areas.

GAO-12-669 VA and DOD Federal Health Care Center Update

Some integration areas cannot be met until a certain point in the integration or depend on other conditions being met. For example, for the integration benchmarks area and the property area, the Executive Agreement specifies that in accordance with NDAA 2010, property transfer may occur upon the earlier of (1) completion of the 15 integration benchmarks or (2) 5 years from the date the Executive Agreement was executed. Thus, the FHCC may address the property integration area prior to the end of the demonstration, in 2015, but it is not required to do so.

FHCC officials also are in the process of addressing other integration areas with provisions that do not have specific deadlines associated with them. For example, for the fiscal authority integration area, FHCC officials continue to make progress implementing the provisions, although they have experienced some challenges. Since our last review, the Joint Fund, into which both VA and DOD contribute, has become operational.[19] However, the provision of the Executive Agreement in the fiscal authority integration area that requires the FHCC to develop an operating plan by month that includes workload data has not yet been met. Specifically, the FHCC's operating plan does not include workload data, which officials reported is because the current VA and DOD IT systems calculate workload data differently. (See table 3.)

[19]The FHCC was not able to operate the Joint Fund until funds had been authorized and appropriated for VA and DOD to transfer into the Joint Fund, which occurred in April 2011. Pub. L. No. 112-10, div. A, § 8107, div. B, §§ 2017, 2018, 125 Stat. 38 (2011).

Table 3: Federal Health Care Center (FHCC) Executive Agreement—Status of Key Provisions of Currently In Progress Integration Areas

Integration area[a]	Status of key provisions as of July 2011[b]	Status of key provisions as of May 2012
Integration benchmarks	Collection of data and assessment of performance on the 15 benchmarks had begun. Benchmarks may be addressed prior to the conclusion of demonstration in 2015.	Past progress maintained by continued collection and assessment of data on the 15 benchmarks to be addressed prior to 2015.
Property	Construction of the facility was completed. Transfer of property to the Department of Veterans Affairs (VA) may occur by completion of demonstration in 2015.	Property transfer provision may be met by completion of demonstration by 2015.
Reporting requirements	VA and the Department of Defense (DOD) required to report to congressional committees following completion of demonstration. This final report is due October 2015.	Provision to report to congressional committees to be met following completion of demonstration in October 2015.
Workforce management and personnel	Provisions related to staffing, training, and the transfer of DOD civilian personnel were met. VA is required to evaluate the extension of collective bargaining rights for the transferred employees by October 2012.	Past progress in staffing, training, and transfer of employees maintained. Provision to evaluate the extension of the collective bargaining rights to be met by October 2012.
Fiscal authority	Developed an integrated budgeting and financial reconciliation process. Developed the Joint DOD-VA Medical Facility Demonstration Fund (Joint Fund) process, but had not implemented it. An automated reconciliation report is to be generated by December 31, 2013, and additional provisions are to be met at a future date.	Joint Fund has been implemented, and past progress of implemented provisions maintained. An automated reconciliation report to be generated by December 31, 2013. An operating plan by month including workload data to be developed.

Source: GAO.

[a]We reported these integration areas as in progress in July 2011; see GAO, *VA and DOD Health Care: First Federal Health Care Center Established, but Implementation Concerns Need to Be Addressed*, GAO-11-570 (Washington, D.C.: July 19, 2011). Two additional integration areas—quality assurance and contingency planning—were in progress at the time of the last report and are now implemented (see table 2).

[b]See GAO-11-570.

GAO-12-669 VA and DOD Federal Health Care Center Update

Continued Delays in the Remaining Executive Agreement Integration Area—IT Implementation—Have Resulted in Additional Costs for the FHCC

Despite some progress, the FHCC continues to face costly delays in the IT integration area. The Executive Agreement specified three key IT capabilities that VA and DOD were required to have in place on opening day, in October 2010, to facilitate interoperability of VA and DOD electronic health record systems.[20] In our 2011 report, we found that all three of these IT components were delayed; some of them continue to remain so. As a result of these delays, the FHCC has had to implement costly workarounds to address the needs these capabilities were intended to serve. In addition to delays in developing these specific IT capabilities, other IT capabilities required by the Executive Agreement have not been well defined and implementation plans for them have not been established.

Specifically, in our 2011 report, we noted that none of the following three IT capabilities required by the Executive Agreement to be in operation by October 2010 were implemented by that time: (1) medical single sign-on, which would allow staff to use one screen to access both the VA and DOD electronic health record systems; (2) single patient registration, which would allow staff to register patients in both systems simultaneously; and (3) orders portability, which would allow VA and DOD clinicians to place, manage, and update clinical orders from either VA or DOD electronic health records systems for radiology, laboratory, consults (specialty referrals), and pharmacy services.

Although none of these capabilities were in place at the time of the FHCC's opening, FHCC officials reported that subsequently, in December 2010, medical single sign-on and single patient registration became operational, as we noted in our 2011 report. Two orders portability components—pharmacy and consults—remain delayed as of May 2012. While orders portability for pharmacy remains delayed, VA and DOD officials have estimated completion of the consults component by March 2013. Since our last review, orders portability for radiology became operational in June 2011 and for laboratory in March 2012. Officials report that as of March 2012, VA and DOD have spent more than $122 million on IT capabilities at the FHCC.

---

[20]VA and DOD rely on separate electronic health record systems to create, maintain, and manage patient health information.

Status of IT Capabilities Required for FHCC

1. Medical single sign-on, which would allow staff to use one screen to access both the Departments of Veterans Affairs (VA) and Defense (DOD) electronic health record systems- required by October 2010, delivered December 2010

2. Single patient registration, which would allow staff to register patients in both systems simultaneously—required by October 2010, delivered December 2010

3. Orders portability, which would allow VA and DOD clinicians to manage clinical orders from either VA or DOD electronic health records systems—four components required by October 2010:

- Pharmacy component delayed

- Consults component not delivered—estimated delivery date March 2013

- Radiology component delivered June 2011

- Laboratory component delivered March 2012

Source: GAO.

VA and DOD officials reported several reasons for the delays in each of the orders portability components and described the workarounds implemented as a result of these delays.

- **Pharmacy component**: Officials have said that they no longer plan to develop a FHCC-specific capability that will allow VA's and DOD's electronic health record systems to exchange information for pharmacy orders, as required by the Executive Agreement, until a more long-term effort to merge the departments' electronic health record systems into a single system is complete. In March 2011, the Secretaries of VA and Defense announced that the two departments had committed to this broader effort, but the departments have not determined when this single electronic health record system will be completed. Officials reported that they have assigned a project team to address this requirement and estimate that they will award a contract for the pharmacy solution by November 2012. Meanwhile, the FHCC continues to maintain the interim orders portability workaround that we previously reported on, which includes five dedicated, full-time pharmacists to conduct manual checks of patient records to reconcile allergy information and identify possible interactions between drugs prescribed in VA and DOD systems. Additionally, FHCC officials reported that they have also hired a full-time pharmacy technician to assist in this process. FHCC officials reported that as of March 2012, they have spent close to $1 million to institute this workaround and that they anticipate spending an additional $750,000 to fund this process from April 2012 through April 2013.

- **Consults component**: VA and DOD officials reported that this component, which will allow VA's and DOD's electronic health record systems to exchange information for consult orders, remains delayed because of changes to the requirements for this component in response to lessons learned since the FHCC opened. Officials reported that they completed the process of documenting changes to the requirements in February 2012 and will use that information to develop the consults component. Until this IT component is implemented, the FHCC staff in the specialty care clinics manage the consult orders manually by reviewing daily all consult requests to determine if care could be provided at the FHCC, in which case the order is manually entered into the appropriate system.

- **Radiology component**: Officials told us that this area was delayed in part because they underestimated the amount of work required to allow VA's and DOD's electronic health record systems to exchange information for radiology orders, and they needed additional time to resolve software defects related to the work.

- **Laboratory component**: Officials reported that there were delays in delivering a capability that would allow the VA and DOD systems to exchange information for laboratory orders because they needed to address software differences between the VA and DOD systems, such as how the systems detect and combine duplicate orders. In addition, they acknowledged that they underestimated the time and effort required to address such differences. Before the laboratory component was implemented, the FHCC instituted a workaround that required health care providers to review both VA and DOD systems for notifications of laboratory results.

Although they were unable to quantify the total cost for all the workarounds resulting from delayed IT capabilities, FHCC officials reported that staff time equivalent to 23 full-time employees is being used to manage the workarounds as a result of delays in IT capabilities to support pharmacy, consults, radiology, and laboratory as well as delays to the other IT components not delivered on time.

In addition to the three delayed IT capabilities that were to be in operation by opening day, implementation of three other IT capabilities required, but not defined, by the Executive Agreement—documentation of patient care to support medical and dental operational readiness, financial management solutions, and outpatient appointment enhancements—also have not been implemented, and in some cases work on them has not begun. The Executive Agreement does not provide clear and specific definitions of these three capabilities, nor does it outline deadlines or specific deliverables. Officials reported that as of May 2012, they had not begun to address the requirements for two of the three capabilities—documentation of patient care to support medical and dental operational readiness and outpatient appointment enhancements—nor had they developed plans or time frames for doing so. VA and DOD officials reported that they have determined the requirements for and have begun the technical development of the financial management solutions, such as automated financial reconciliation and billing processes, and they estimate that testing of the initial capability for the financial reconciliation requirement will occur in July 2012.

Lack of an MTF Designation for the FHCC Continues to Pose Implementation Challenges

FHCC officials continue to experience implementation challenges related to the FHCC's lack of an MTF designation. In our July 2011 report, we noted several challenges associated with the lack of an MTF designation at the FHCC, including limits on its ability to access DOD's drug pricing arrangements for DOD beneficiaries and to use personal services contracts to meet staffing needs, as had been done by DOD prior to the integration.[21] As a result, we recommended that DOD seek a legislative change to designate the FHCC as an MTF to facilitate sharing of all DOD authorities and privileges for the facility. Although DOD concurred with our assessment of challenges based on the lack of an MTF designation, the department has opted not to pursue our recommendation. DOD stated that it anticipates that as the FHCC stabilizes and matures, the confusion caused by the lack of an MTF designation will dissipate and that the challenges we noted in the last report have been addressed by workarounds. However, we have found that some of the integration implementation challenges that could be solved with such a designation remain. In particular, officials told us the FHCC has been denied access to DOD's drug pricing arrangements for its DOD beneficiaries, which has resulted in the FHCC paying higher prices for certain drugs for DOD beneficiaries than would be the case if it were an MTF, although FHCC officials were unable to quantify the added expense. DOD officials told us

---

[21]See GAO-11-570.

that the department continues to explore ways to access DOD's drug pricing arrangements, despite the lack of an MTF designation, but that so far these efforts have not been successful. In addition, FHCC officials have instituted a workaround to enable them to fulfill staffing needs using personal services contracts—a preferred method for accommodating fluctuations in medical and dental workloads resulting from increases in the number of Navy recruits on-site at any given time.[22] If the FHCC was designated as an MTF, it would have the authority to use personal services contracts, making such a workaround unnecessary. We continue to believe that an MTF designation is important to address the challenges the FHCC faces based on the lack of such a designation, and because it would set a precedent for future VA and DOD integrations to help make the integration process smoother.

VA and DOD Have Not Yet Established a Plan for Evaluating the FHCC Demonstration

Although they are required by NDAA 2010 to conduct a comprehensive evaluation of the FHCC at the end of the 5-year demonstration and submit a report on this evaluation to the House and Senate Committees on Armed Services and Veterans' Affairs, VA and DOD officials said the departments have not yet established an evaluation plan. We have previously found that developing a sound evaluation plan before a demonstration program is implemented can increase confidence in results and facilitate decision making about broader applications of the demonstration.[23] Without such a plan in place during the demonstration—including well-defined measures and standards, such as target scores, for determining performance on each measure—FHCC leadership cannot track progress and make adjustments to improve performance in areas that VA and DOD determine are necessary for the FHCC's success.[24] In addition, we have previously found that joint agreement on commonly desired outcomes, such as those established as performance measures and standards in an evaluation plan, is important for collaborating agencies, such as VA and DOD, to successfully overcome differences in

---

[22]The FHCC processes nearly 40,000 Navy recruits each year, ensuring that each recruit is medically ready for service.

[23]GAO-08-387R and GAO-09-45.

[24]GAO-09-45.

their agency missions, cultures, and established ways of doing business.[25]

VA and DOD officials told us that at the end of the demonstration, they expect the FHCC Advisory Board, along with the HEC and JEC—the governing bodies that provide executive oversight for VA and DOD collaborations—to assess the demonstration and provide recommendations to the departments about whether the FHCC should continue. These assessments will inform the Secretaries of VA and Defense, who will ultimately issue a report and recommendation to congressional committees regarding the FHCC. Officials confirmed that they will use the 15 integration benchmarks established in the Executive Agreement as part of the assessment (see app. I),[26] which as we previously reported, are monitored and reported by FHCC officials using a FHCC-developed tool.[27] In addition to these benchmarks, VA and DOD officials also have said they expect to consider additional factors, which may include performance measures, in evaluating the FHCC's performance at the end of the demonstration. Officials explained that the 15 integration benchmarks do not address all factors relevant to determining the FHCC's utility as an integrated model for delivering health care. Among the additional factors DOD and VA officials say they are considering are the following:

- an Institute of Medicine study commissioned by DOD to determine whether the quality of, and access to, services provided by the

---

[25]GAO, *Results-Oriented Government: Practices That Can Help Enhance and Sustain Collaboration among Federal Agencies*, GAO-06-15 (Washington, D.C.: Oct. 21, 2005).

[26]The 15 integration benchmarks comprise 38 individual performance measures. For example, the patient satisfaction benchmark is measured using 2 performance measures—a VA measure and a DOD measure based on separate surveys that assess beneficiaries' experience with care at the FHCC.

[27]In response to a recommendation we made in our July 2011 report, FHCC officials have made changes to this tool. Specifically, we raised concerns regarding the accuracy and transparency of the information generated by this reporting tool and also about the ability of FHCC's use of a single monthly summary score to provide a meaningful gauge of success. We were particularly concerned about the use of this summary score given that VA and DOD had not established specific targets to define success. In response to our concerns, officials have (1) corrected a calculation error to make the summary score more accurate and (2) altered their methodology to ensure that the summary score better reflects performance rather than fluctuations caused by varied data collection time frames, as had occurred previously. See GAO-11-570.

integrated FHCC meet or exceed those of NCVAMC and NHCGL as separate facilities prior to the integration;[28]

- an evaluation of whether the services available at the FHCC are appropriate for the needs of its beneficiary population (for example, whether the pediatrics workload is sufficient to maintain a pediatrics department at the FHCC or whether it would be more cost-effective to contract for pediatrics care in the local community);

- personnel-related factors, such as whether corpsmen are able to be used at their full capacity at the FHCC and develop the medical skills needed for deployment;[29] and

- FHCC costs.

Furthermore, VA and DOD have not set specific target scores for determining successful performance for the existing 15 integration benchmarks. Officials told us they do not expect to establish these scores until the end of the 5-year FHCC demonstration.

Although federal financial accounting standards, VA and DOD departmental priorities, and the Executive Agreement—which lays out the purpose of the FHCC—indicate that reliable cost information is important for evaluating the FHCC, VA and DOD officials have not determined what cost measures, if any, will be used in the FHCC's evaluation. In particular, federal financial accounting standards state that Congress and federal executives need reliable cost information to compare alternative courses of action and evaluate program performance.[30] In addition, both the Veterans Health Administration's vision statement and the Military Health System's core values statement highlight the importance of cost or value of health care to VA and DOD. Furthermore, VA and DOD jointly agreed through the Executive Agreement that the FHCC itself was designed to

---

[28]The Institute of Medicine expects to publish the results of this study in the fall of 2012.

[29]Officials explained that corpsmen—enlisted personnel who receive advanced training to provide treatment and administer medications—must be able to fully develop skills at the FHCC that they will need to be ready for service in the field when deployed, such as medical skills needed in combat areas.

[30]Federal Accounting Standards Advisory Board, *Statement of Federal Financial Accounting Standards 4: Managerial Cost Accounting Standards and Concepts* (Washington, D.C.: July 1995).

improve cost-effectiveness of health care delivery, along with access and quality, for the beneficiaries of NHCGL and NCVAMC. Prior to the integration, FHCC officials reported that cost savings, mainly one-time construction savings, were one of the original considerations in deciding to integrate the two facilities, but FHCC officials told us that they are unable to determine whether these savings were actually realized.[31] We have previously reported that cost-effectiveness information is important for ensuring that a program produces sufficient benefits in relation to its costs.[32] Although the existing FHCC integration benchmarks include measures related to access and quality, they do not include any measures related to cost-effectiveness, and while VA and DOD officials said they are considering incorporating cost into the evaluation, they still have not determined whether to do so or what cost measures will be used.

Conclusions

The FHCC is a 5-year demonstration that has the potential to be a model for future VA and DOD collaborations to deliver high-quality and cost-effective integrated health care services. However, the demonstration has notable problems. The lack of an MTF designation; costly delays in IT implementation and the lack of clear definitions, deliverables, and time frames for certain IT capabilities; and the lack of an overall evaluation plan for the demonstration pose challenges to VA, DOD, and FHCC officials.

Because the FHCC does not have an MTF designation, FHCC officials continue to experience additional costs and administrative burden. The FHCC is unable to use DOD drug pricing arrangements for DOD beneficiaries, which has resulted in additional costs for the FHCC, and also cannot use personal services contracts without the need for a workaround. Because of these ongoing problems, we continue to believe

---

[31]In a 2009 report, FHCC officials projected that the integration would result in one-time cost savings of $67 million by avoiding the need to build a new naval hospital and recurring annual cost savings of $22.3 million by reducing operating costs and staff size when compared to the projected costs for NCVAMC and NHCGL separately. They have contracted with the Center for Naval Analyses to conduct an assessment of the costs associated with the FHCC's integration, including past and current costs through the early stages of the demonstration. This assessment is also intended to document any cost savings associated with FHCC patient care.

[32]GAO-09-45.

that the Secretary of Defense should seek a legislative change to designate the FHCC as an MTF, even if only for the period of the 5-year demonstration.

Delays in the implementation of key IT components required by the Executive Agreement to be in place by October 2010 have resulted in the FHCC establishing workarounds in an effort to maintain patient care and safety. In some cases, these workarounds have been costly and inefficient, necessitating the hiring of additional staff or using additional staff time to do manually what the IT systems are intended to automate. After spending more than $122 million on IT capabilities needed for the FHCC, key deliverables remain delayed, resulting in additional costs to the FHCC. For example, officials have spent more than $1 million as of May 2012 on workarounds for the pharmacy component alone, with an additional $750,000 of spending expected through April 2013. Having a clear understanding of the costs associated with workarounds needed when IT systems are not in place is essential in planning any future VA and DOD integration efforts. In addition, the lack of clarity for time frames and deliverables for two other IT requirements included in the Executive Agreement may pose challenges for implementing them during the demonstration.

Despite the fact that the demonstration is in its second of 5 years, DOD and VA have yet to develop and implement an overall evaluation plan. Without such a plan, decision makers at all levels lack the information needed to evaluate the FHCC in a transparent way that ensures confidence in the results. Establishing an evaluation plan, including relevant measures and standards, such as target scores for the benchmarks, as early as possible during the demonstration also provides FHCC officials the opportunity to make informed midcourse changes to better ensure the delivery of high-quality and cost-effective care. It also will better facilitate decision making about whether replicating the model in other locations is prudent. Finally, without assessing the cost-effectiveness of the FHCC, VA and DOD decision makers, as well as Congress, will be unable to adequately assess whether the integrated health care delivery model of the FHCC produces sufficient benefits in relation to its costs.

Recommendations for Executive Action

To clarify IT requirements within the Executive Agreement, to enable VA and DOD to make an informed recommendation about whether the FHCC should continue after the end of the demonstration, and to provide useful information for other integrations that may be considered in the future, we recommend that the Secretaries of Veterans Affairs and Defense take the following four actions:

- determine the costs associated with the workarounds required because of delayed IT capabilities at the FHCC for each year of the demonstration, including the costs of hiring additional staff and of managing the administrative burden caused by the workarounds;

- develop plans with clear definitions and specific deliverables, including time frames for two IT capabilities—documentation of patient care to support medical and dental operational readiness and outpatient appointment enhancements—and formalize these plans, for example, by incorporating them into the Executive Agreement;

- expeditiously develop and agree to an evaluation plan, including the performance measures and standards, such as target scores, to be used to evaluate the FHCC demonstration, and formalize the plan, for example, by incorporating it into the Executive Agreement; and

- establish measures related to the cost-effectiveness of the FHCC's care and operations to be included as a part of the evaluation plan.

Agency Comments and Our Evaluation

DOD and VA each provided comments on a draft of this report. In their comments, both agencies generally concurred with each of the four recommendations to the Secretaries of Defense and Veterans Affairs. (DOD's comments are reprinted in app. II; VA's comments are reprinted in app. III.) In addition, both VA and DOD provided technical comments which we have incorporated as appropriate. The agencies' specific responses to each of our recommendations are as follows:

- To determine the costs associated with the workarounds required because of delayed IT capabilities at the FHCC, DOD indicated that it will collaborate with VA to determine these costs. VA stated the FHCC will convene a workgroup to review these costs and to identify any additional needs associated with IT development delays. VA suggested changing "workaround" to "impacts and changes to business practices." We maintain that "workaround" is used appropriately in the context of this report because we use it to describe processes that are temporarily in place for the purpose of mitigating IT delays rather than permanent changes to business practices.

- To develop plans with clear definitions and specific deliverables, including time frames for two IT capabilities, both VA and DOD stated that they are working together through their joint Interagency Program Office to develop and formalize these plans. DOD added that the Interagency Program Office will also consider how these plans relate to the larger effort to implement an integrated electronic health record. Both agencies noted that formalization of these plans does not require incorporation into the Executive Agreement. We offered amending the Executive Agreement as an example of how plans could be formalized and leave it to the agencies' discretion how best to do so.

- To expeditiously develop and agree to an evaluation plan, VA and DOD mentioned that although a methodology and framework for a final evaluation have not been determined, they are tracking some measures of performance through the 15 integration benchmarks. In addition, VA stated that the JEC has directed the HEC to outline an evaluation plan to include analysis of personnel, logistics, resources, and regulatory issues. Again, both agencies noted that formalizing of the evaluation plan does not require incorporation into the Executive Agreement. As we noted above, amending the Executive Agreement is one option for how the plan could be formalized and the agencies may determine the most effective way to do so.

- To establish measures related to the cost-effectiveness of the FHCC's care and operations to be included as a part of the evaluation plan, VA stated that it will develop a process to expedite creation of an evaluation plan. Both agencies concurred with the recommendation to include cost-related measures.

VA provided an additional comment regarding the issue of MTF designation at the FHCC. They suggest that VA and DOD agree on the matter of seeking an MTF designation before any action is taken regarding establishing the FHCC as an MTF.

We are sending copies of this report to the Secretary of Defense, Secretary of Veterans Affairs, and appropriate congressional committees. In addition, the report is available at no charge on the GAO website at http://www.gao.gov.

If you or your staff have any questions about this report, please contact me at (202) 512-7114 or draperd@gao.gov. Contact points for our Offices of Congressional Relations and Public Affairs may be found on the last page of this report. GAO staff who made major contributions to this report are listed in appendix IV.

Debra A. Draper
Director, Health Care

List of Committees

The Honorable Carl Levin
Chairman
The Honorable John S. McCain
Ranking Member
Committee on Armed Services
United States Senate

The Honorable Patty Murray
Chairman
The Honorable Richard Burr
Ranking Member
Committee on Veterans' Affairs
United States Senate

The Honorable Howard P. "Buck" McKeon
Chairman
The Honorable Adam Smith
Ranking Member
Committee on Armed Services
House of Representatives

The Honorable Jeff Miller
Chairman
The Honorable Bob Filner
Ranking Member
Committee on Veterans' Affairs
House of Representatives

Appendix I: Federal Health Care Center Integration Benchmarks, by Number of Reported Measures

Integration benchmarks	Number of individual performance measures to be reported
1. Patient satisfaction measures meet Federal Health Care Center (FHCC) targets.	2
2. Staff surveys meet FHCC targets.	2
3. Health profession trainee satisfaction measures meet FHCC targets.	1
4. Stakeholders Advisory Council determination that the FHCC meets both Department of Veterans Affairs (VA) and Department of Defense (DOD) missions.[a]	1
5. Clinical and administrative performance measures meet FHCC targets.	4
6. Patient access to care meets FHCC targets.	3
7. Evidence-based health care measures meet FHCC targets.	2
8. Clinical/dental productivity meets FHCC targets.	3
9. Information technology solution timeline is met and has no negative impact on patient safety.	1
10. Pre-FHCC academic and clinical research missions are maintained.	2
11. Navy servicemember medical readiness for duty meets Navy targets.	3
12. Navy advancement/retention meets Navy targets.	3
13. Successful annual GAO review.	1
14. Validation of FHCC fiscal reconciliation model by an annual independent audit.	1
15. Satisfactory facility and clinical inspection, accreditation, and compliance outcomes from several external oversight/groups, such as VA and DOD Offices of the Inspector General and The Joint Commission.[b]	9
Total	**38**

Source: GAO.

[a]The Stakeholders Advisory Council is composed of members from various organizations representing FHCC interests, including a local government representative, as well as officials from TRICARE and nearby VA medical facilities located in Hines, Illinois, and Milwaukee, Wisconsin. It provides feedback on how well the FHCC is meeting customers' needs and whether the FHCC is meeting VA and DOD missions.

[b]The Joint Commission is an independent organization that accredits and certifies health care organizations and programs in the United States.

Appendix II: Comments from the Department of Defense

Note: GAO received DOD's letter commenting on a draft of this report on June 11, 2012.

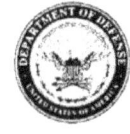

THE ASSISTANT SECRETARY OF DEFENSE

1200 DEFENSE PENTAGON
WASHINGTON, DC 20301-1200

HEALTH AFFAIRS

Ms. Debra Draper
Director, Health Care
U.S. Government Accountability Office
441 G Street, NW
Washington, DC 20548

Dear Ms. Draper:

This is the Department of Defense's (DoD) response to the Government Accountability Office's (GAO) draft report GAO-12-669, "VA/DOD FEDERAL HEALTH CARE CENTER: Costly Information Technology Delays Continue and Evaluation Plan Lacking," dated May 11, 2012 (GAO Code - 290987). The Department appreciates the opportunity to comment on the draft report.

The Department generally concurs with each of the four recommendations. Also enclosed are specific, technical comments regarding details contained in the body of the report that the Department believes will add clarity and some instances of improved accuracy.

Please direct any questions to the points of contact on this matter, Mr. Kenneth E. Cox (Functional) and Mr. Gunther J. Zimmerman (Audit Liaison). Mr. Cox may be reached at (703) 681-4258, or Kenneth.Cox@tma.osd.mil. Mr. Zimmerman may be reached at (703) 681-3492, ext. 4065, or Gunther.Zimmerman@tma.osd.mil.

Sincerely,

Jonathan Woodson, M.D.

Enclosures:
1. Overall Comments
2. Technical Comments
3. Interagency Program Office Comments
4. Department of the Navy Comments

GOVERNMENT ACCOUNTABILITY OFFICE
DRAFT REPORT – DATED MAY 11, 2011
(GAO CODE - 290987)

"VA/DOD FEDERAL HEALTH CARE CENTER: Costly Information Technology Delays
Continue and Evaluation Plan Lacking"

DEPARTMENT OF DEFENSE COMMENTS

RECOMMENDATION 1: The GAO recommends that the Secretaries of Veterans Affairs
(VA) and Defense determine the costs associated with the workarounds required due to delayed
Information Technology (IT) capabilities at the Federal Health Care Center (FHCC) for each
year of the demonstration, including the costs of hiring additional staff and of managing the
administrative burden due to workarounds.

DoD RESPONSE: The Department of Defense (DoD) concurs with the recommendation to
determine the costs associated with workarounds required as a result of delays in the
implementation of specific IT capabilities at the James A. Lovell FHCC. The costs associated
with the Orders Portability Pharmacy workaround are documented in the GAO's report, but DoD
will collaborate with VA to determine the cost of other IT workarounds, if any.

RECOMMENDATION 2: The GAO recommends that the Secretaries of VA and DoD
develop plans with clear definitions and specific deliverables including timeframes for two IT
capabilities—documentation of patient care to support medical and dental operational readiness
and outpatient appointment enhancements—and formalize these plans such as by incorporating
them into the Executive Agreement for the DoD-VA Medical Facility Demonstration Project at
the FHCC.

DoD RESPONSE: DoD concurs with the recommendation to develop plans with clear
definition and specific deliverables for the two IT capabilities and formalize these plans.
Consistent with its charter, the VA/DoD Interagency Program Office (IPO) is working with DoD
and VA to develop and formalize plans with clear definitions and specific deliverables including
timeframes for two IT capabilities (documentation of patient care to support medical and dental
operational readiness and outpatient appointment enhancements). Formalization of these plans
does not require incorporation into the Executive Agreement.

Additionally, IPO will work with VA (Office of Information and Technology and the Veterans
Health Administration), DoD, and FHCC Officials to develop plans with clear definitions,
specifications, deliverables, and timeframes for IT capabilities and how those plans relate to the
integrated electronic health record (iEHR) effort. The anticipated completion date is December
2012.

Finally, as it was previously reported, it is anticipated that FHCC products will support
documentation of patient care with regard to medical and dental operational readiness, and
functional representatives will assess this capability as the work environment evolves at FHCC.

See responses to GAO's Question #2 received January 25, 2012, and Question #6 received February 24, 2012.

RECOMMENDATION 3: The GAO recommends that the Secretaries of VA and DoD expeditiously develop and agree to an evaluation plan, including the performance measures and standards, such as target scores, to be used to evaluate the FHCC's demonstration, and formalize the plan, such as by incorporating them into the Executive Agreement.

DoD RESPONSE: DoD concurs with the recommendation to develop an evaluation plan and to formalize that plan. Formalization of this plan does not require incorporation into the Executive Agreement.

The Executive Agreement states: The Navy Bureau of Medicine and Surgery (BUMED), Navy Medicine East, and VA have agreed on Benchmarks to define the degree of integration success (Section VI, J). Attachment A Section 7 (below) lists the Benchmarks.

The FHCC established the baseline for these measures prior to integration and established control limits for each measure. FHCC staff evaluate each month whether the measures are better, worse, or unchanged since enacting the Executive Agreement.

Additionally, DoD has contracted with the Institute of Medicine (IOM) to study the collaboration efforts at the FHCC. The IOM will evaluate whether the integrated DoD and Veterans Administration health care facility in North Chicago is more beneficial to DoD and VA in serving the needs of their eligible populations than their independent facilities. DoD and VA are engaged in efforts to determine lessons learned and cultural integration with the assistance of the VA National Center for Organizational Development.

Finally, while a framework and methodology for the final evaluation and report have not been determined, there are currently evaluation criteria in place and on-going in the following areas:

1. Patient satisfaction measures meet VA and DoD benchmarks.
2. Maintenance of Medical Individual Accounts for Recruits at less than five percent; maintain Training Center Support Students Not Under Instruction for medical reasons at less than two percent; Individual Medical Readiness — indeterminate status for active duty less than five percent.
3. Stakeholders Advisory Council determination that the FHCC meets both DoD and VA missions.
4. Successful annual Comptroller General review.
5. Validation of fiscal reconciliation report by annual independent audit.
6. VA clinical and administrative performance measures exceed mean for all VA Medical Centers.
7. Meet all access to care standards.
8. Evidence-Based Health Care measures meet or exceed VA and DoD mean.
9. Satisfactory clinical and facility inspection outcomes from external oversight/accreditation groups, including but not limited to:
   a. Joint Commission

    b. VA Office of Inspector General (OIG)

    c. DoD OIG

    d. VA Office of the Medical Inspector

    e. BUMED Medical Inspector General

    f. American Association of Blood Banks

    g. Food and Drug Administration

    h. College of American Pathologists

    i. Occupational Safety and Health Administration

10. Officer promotion/retention and enlisted advancement/retention meet or exceed Department of Navy means.

11. Information Management (IM)/IT implementation timeline met and no negative impact on patient safety.

12. Staff satisfaction and other appropriate measures identified as VA and DoD benchmarks.

13. Relative Value Unit/Relative Weighted Product/Dental Weighted Value production meets Business Plan targets.

14. Maintain pre-FHCC academic and clinical research missions.

15. Trainee Satisfaction as measured by the Learner Perception Survey.

RECOMMENDATION 4: The GAO recommends that the Secretaries of VA and DoD establish measures related to the cost-effectiveness of the FHCC's care and operations to be included as a part of the evaluation plan.

DoD RESPONSE: DoD concurs with the recommendation to include cost-effectiveness measures in the evaluation plan.

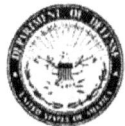

DEPARTMENT OF THE NAVY
BUREAU OF MEDICINE AND SURGERY

6010
M3/E12UN093-000570

JUN 1 1 2012

MEMORANDUM FOR ASSISTANT SECRETARY OF DEFENSE (HEALTH AFFAIRS)

SUBJECT: Draft Report on VA/DoD Federal Health Care Center: Costly Information
Technology Delays Continue and Evaluation Plan Lacking dated May 2012
(GAO Code 290987)

Thank you for the opportunity to review and comment on the GAO Draft Report on
VA/DoD Federal Health Care Center: Costly Information Technology Delays Continue and
Evaluation Plan Lacking dated May 2012. Navy Medicine generally concurs with each of the
four recommendations; however we do not agree that the detailed Information Technology and
Evaluation Plans require incorporation into the Executive Agreement to ensure their execution.
Enclosed are comments as requested regarding details contained in the draft report.

My point of contact for this matter is Ms. Tamara Rollins at (202) 762-3520 or
Tamara.Rollins@med.navy.mil.

D. L. STYLES
Deputy Chief, Medical Operations
Acting

Attachments:
As stated

GOVERNMENT ACCOUNTABILITY OFFICE

DRAFT REPORT (GAO CODE - 290987) – DATED MAY 18, 2011

"VA/DOD FEDERAL HEALTH CARE CENTER: Costly Information Technology Delays
Continue and Evaluation Plan Lacking"

<u>NAVY MEDICINE COMMENTS</u>

RECOMMENDATION 1: The Government Accountability Office (GAO) recommends the
Secretaries of Defense and Veterans Affairs determine the costs associated with the workarounds
required due to delayed IT capabilities at the FHCC for each year of the demonstration, including
the costs of hiring additional staff and of managing the administrative burden due to
workarounds.

NAVY RESPONSE: Navy Medicine concurs with the recommendation to determine the costs
associated with workarounds required as a result of delays in the implementation of specific IT
capabilities at the FHCC. The costs associated with the Orders Portability Pharmacy
workaround are documented in the GAO's report.

RECOMMENDATION 2: GAO recommends that the Secretaries of Defense and Veteran
Affairs develop plans with clear definitions and specific deliverables including timeframes for
two IT capabilities—documentation of patient care to support medical and dental operational
readiness and outpatient appointment enhancements—and formalize these plans such as by
incorporating them into the Executive Agreement.

NAVY RESPONSE: Navy Medicine concurs with the recommendation to develop plans with
clear definition and specific deliverables for the two IT capabilities; however we do not concur
that this plan needs to be incorporated into the Executive Agreement.

RECOMMENDATION 3: GAO recommends that the Secretaries of Defense and Veteran
Affairs expeditiously develop and agree to an evaluation plan, including the performance
measures and standards, such as target scores, to be used to evaluate the FHCC demonstration,
and formalize the plan, such as by incorporating them into the Executive Agreement.

NAVY RESPONSE: Navy Medicine concurs with the recommendation to develop an
evaluation plan, however does not concur that the detailed evaluation warrant being added into
the Executive Agreement.

The Executive Agreement states: BUMED, Navy Medicine East, and VA have agreed on
Benchmarks to define the degree of integration success (Section VI, J).

The FHCC established the baseline for these measures prior to integration and established
control limits for each measure. FHCC staff review the measures monthly and evaluate each to
determine whether the measures are better, worse or unchanged since enacting the Executive
Agreement.

1

The Institute of Medicine (IOM) has also been contracted by OASD/HA to study the collaboration efforts at the FHCC. The IOM will evaluate whether the integrated Department of Defense and Veterans Administration (DoD/VA) health care facility in North Chicago is more beneficial to DoD and VA in serving the needs of their eligible populations than their independent facilities.

RECOMMENDATION 4: GAO recommends that the Secretaries of Defense and Veteran Affairs establish measures related to the cost-effectiveness of the FHCC's care and operations to be included as part of the evaluation plan.

NAVY RESPONSE: Navy Medicine concurs with the recommendation to include cost-effectiveness measures in the evaluation plan.

2

Appendix III: Comments from the Department of Veterans Affairs

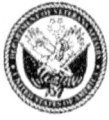

DEPARTMENT OF VETERANS AFFAIRS
WASHINGTON DC 20420

June 11, 2012

Ms. Debra Draper
Director, Health Care
U.S. Government Accountability Office
441 G Street, NW
Washington, DC 20548

Dear Ms. Draper:

The Department of Veterans Affairs (VA) has reviewed the Government Accountability Office's (GAO) draft report, *"VA/DOD FEDERAL HEALTH CARE CENTER: Costly Information Technology Delays Continue and Evaluation Plan Lacking"* (GAO-12-669) and generally concurs with GAO's four recommendations to the Department.

The enclosure specifically addresses GAO's four recommendations and provides an action plan for each and provides general and technical comments. VA appreciates the opportunity to comment on your draft report.

Sincerely,

John R. Gingrich
Chief of Staff

Enclosures

Enclosure

Department of Veterans Affairs (VA) Comments to
Government Accountability Office (GAO) Draft Report:
*VA/DOD FEDERAL HEALTH CARE CENTER: Costly Information
Technology Delays Continue and Evaluation Plan Lacking*
(GAO-12-669)

GAO Recommendation: To clarify IT requirements within the Executive Agreement, to
enable VA and DOD to make an informed decision about whether the FHCC should
continue after the end of the demonstration, and to provide useful information for other
integrations that may be considered in the future, we recommend the Secretaries of
Veterans Affairs and Defense take the following four actions:

Recommendation 1: determine the costs associated with the workarounds required
due to delayed IT capabilities at the FHCC for each year of the demonstration, including
the costs of hiring additional staff and of managing the administrative burden to
workarounds.

VA Response: Concur with comments. The Veterans Health Administration (VHA)
suggests that the GAO not use the term "workarounds" and instead refer to what the
Federal Health Care Center (FHCC) has implemented as "impacts and changes to
business practices." The term workaround is an incomplete portrayal of the efforts VA
has made. Addressing what business practices were changed and the impact of these
changes ensures a more complete and accurate capture of the costs of delaying IT
capabilities.

VA concurs with the recommendation to determine the costs associated with the
impacts and changes to business practices due to delayed information technology (IT)
development and the operational impact of testing and deploying new IT solutions. As
noted in the GAO draft report on pages 16 and 17, the FHCC has already allocated
additional funding to support staff needed for the pharmacy and laboratory processes
due to delays in IT development. The need for these staff was determined by a
multidisciplinary group, who focused on how to ensure patient safety without the
integrated record. Also, the FHCC has dedicated approximately 23 full-time equivalents
(FTE) to support the operational impacts, as stated in the report. The FHCC will
maintain the additional resources at the site until the IT solutions are in place and
discussions are underway with the VHA Chief Financial Officer (CFO) and the
Department of Navy's (DON) Bureau of Medicine and Surgery (BUMED) Comptroller to
determine how funding for these resources will be addressed.

Because the total costs of the impacts and changes to business practices have not
been tracked previously and to ensure that all potential liabilities associated with IT
delays are identified, the FHCC will convene a workgroup under the authority of the
FHCC Advisory Board. The workgroup will consist of appropriate subject matter experts
(SME) as well as front line clinicians to identify any further gaps that may exist beyond
the pharmacy and laboratory arenas associated with IT development delays and
operational impacts, focusing on what needs to be done to ensure patient safety. The

1

Enclosure

Department of Veterans Affairs (VA) Comments to
Government Accountability Office (GAO) Draft Report:
*VA/DOD FEDERAL HEALTH CARE CENTER: Costly Information
Technology Delays Continue and Evaluation Plan Lacking*
(GAO-12-669)

workgroup will also review and validate the total costs of implementing changes to business practices as determined and tracked by the FHCC. The FHCC Advisory Board will report to the Health Executive Committee (HEC) no later than December 31, 2012, and will provide a plan on the level of additional staff required by the FHCC, as well as a plan for funding that staff.

Recommendation 2: develop plans with clear definitions and specific deliverables including timeframes for two IT capabilities—documentation of patient care to support medical and dental operational readiness and outpatient appointment enhancements— and formalize these plans such as by incorporating them into the Executive Agreement.

VA Response: VA concurs with the recommendation to develop plans with clear definition and specific deliverables for the two IT capabilities; however, VA does not concur that this plan needs to be incorporated into the Executive Agreement (EA). Consistent with its charter, the Interagency Program Office (IPO) is working with Department of Defense (DoD) and VA to develop and formalize plans with clear definitions and specific deliverables, including timeframes for two IT capabilities (documentation of patient care to support medical and dental operational readiness and outpatient appointment enhancements). The anticipated completion date is December 2012.

Recommendation 3: expeditiously develop and agree to an evaluation plan, including the performance measures and standards, such as target scores, to be used to evaluate the FHCC demonstration, and formalize the plan, such as incorporating it into the Executive Agreement.

VA Response: VA concurs with the recommendation to expeditiously develop and agree to an evaluation plan however, VA does not concur that this plan needs to be incorporated into the EA. It is important to note that the FHCC EA includes benchmarks to define the degree of integration success (Section VI, J, Attachment A, Section 7). These benchmarks are included as Attachment A of this action plan.

The FHCC established the baseline for these measures prior to integration and established control limits for each measure. FHCC staff evaluates these measures monthly to determine whether the results are better, worse, or unchanged since enacting the EA.

In addition to these benchmark reviews, DoD has contracted with the Institute of Medicine to study the collaboration efforts at the FHCC. With assistance from VA's National Center for Organizational Development, DoD and VA are identifying lessons learned from the organizational and cultural integration.

2

Enclosure

Department of Veterans Affairs (VA) Comments to
Government Accountability Office (GAO) Draft Report:
*VA/DOD FEDERAL HEALTH CARE CENTER: Costly Information
Technology Delays Continue and Evaluation Plan Lacking*
(GAO-12-669)

While a framework and methodology for the final evaluation and report have not been determined, there are currently evaluation criteria in place, and on-going efforts continue. It is also important to note that because this is a demonstration pilot, VA and DoD have been gathering important data and information about topics that were not identified or anticipated at the start of the project. This dynamic process has required flexibility, mindfulness, and agility in order to recognize issues and react effectively. The opportunity to react quickly has been important in order to gather valuable insights about how to successfully establish an integrated facility. These additional lessons learned may include areas such as culture, governance, and new business practices.

In addition to this ongoing context for evaluation, the VA/DoD Joint Executive Committee (JEC) has directed the VA/DoD Health Executive Council (HEC) to prepare the outline for an evaluation plan that will be used to develop the recommendations for the report to Congress. The plan will identify and analyze those personnel, logistics, resourcing, and regulatory issues that apply to FHCC and will be used to assist the Secretaries in making decisions concerning similar future integrated facilities.

Recommendation 4: establish measures related to the cost-effectiveness of the FHCC's care and operations to be inlcuded as a part of the evaluation plan.

VA Response: Concur with comment. VA will develop a process involving VHA, the FHCC, and the VA Office of Policy and Planning to expedite developing and establishing a more formalized evaluation plan.

3

Enclosure

Department of Veterans Affairs (VA) Comments to
Government Accountability Office (GAO) Draft Report:
*VA/DOD FEDERAL HEALTH CARE CENTER: Costly Information
Technology Delays Continue and Evaluation Plan Lacking*
(GAO-12-669)

<u>General Comments</u>

Page 12, paragraph 3: Fiscal Issues/Workload Data: GAO indicates that the
operating plan does not include workload data. The following outlines how the FHCC is
collecting and using these data.

- The FHCC budget call workbooks (Attachment B) reflect that workload data is
  being captured and reported in VA's Decision Support System. These data are
  then used in determining budget amounts. Unfortunately, the FHCC only had
  one year of data to work with for the fiscal year (FY) 2013 budget call. Because
  this budget submission is so early in the year, the FHCC cannot capture the
  previous year workload data. FY 2011 was the base year. The FY 2014 budget
  call workbooks will reflect two years of workload data. In the future, more
  workload data will be available for analysis and to assist in the budgeting
  process.

- GAO's report says that the FHCC's "operating plan does not include workload
  data." This is true from the perspective that the operating plan only requires the
  FHCC to report dollars needed each month to operate the facility. While neither
  the Navy nor VA's operating plan requires workload data be reported, the dollars
  reported on the operating plans do include an analysis of the workload data as
  described previously.

Page 16, Consults Component: The business requirements document for consults
was updated in February 2012 to reflect a year's worth of lessons learned and to
incorporate local changes to the business process as a result of those lessons learned.
The consults IT project is scheduled to deliver its first customer-facing capability in
August 2012, (orders) and finish in February 2013 (results).

Page 16, Radiology and Laboratory Components: Originally the radiology and
laboratory orders portability issues were being worked as one project. It soon became
apparent that the laboratory orders portability was much more complicated than the
radiology orders portability, and the mapping of laboratory orders and results between
electronic health records was a massive under taking. The local leadership decided to
focus on radiology because the daily work load was much lighter for radiology
compared to the laboratory, e.g. processing counts are 500 radiology orders vice
10,000 laboratory orders per day. Radiology was delivered in June 2011. The
technology used to develop the radiology solution was then leveraged to build the
laboratory solution.

4

Enclosure

Department of Veterans Affairs (VA) Comments to
Government Accountability Office (GAO) Draft Report:
*VA/DOD FEDERAL HEALTH CARE CENTER: Costly Information
Technology Delays Continue and Evaluation Plan Lacking*
(GAO-12-669)

Page 17, Military Treatment Facility: The report states that, "Lack of an MTF
designation for the FHCC continues to pose implementation challenges." GAO
provides examples about access to DOD's drug pricing and use of personal
service contracts. Although GAO indicates that a military treatment facility
(MTF) designation is important to address the challenges the FHCC faces and
would set a precedent for future VA and DOD integration to help make the
integration process smoother,

VA suggests that no action regarding a military treatment facility designation
occur without a joint agreement between the Department of Veterans Affairs
and the Department of Defense.

5

ATTACHMENT A

INTEGRATION BENCHMARKS (Executive Agreement, Attachment A, Section 7)

1. Patient satisfaction measures meet Department of Veterans Affairs (VA) and Department of Defense (DoD) benchmarks.
2. Maintenance of Medical Individual Accounts for Recruits at less than five percent; maintain Training Center Support Students Not Under Instruction for medical reasons at less than two percent; Individual Medical Readiness — indeterminate status for active duty less than five percent.
3. Stakeholders Advisory Council (SAC) determination that the Federal Health Care Center (FHCC) meets both DoD and VA missions.
4. Successful annual Comptroller General review.
5. Validation of fiscal reconciliation report by annual independent audit.
6. VA clinical and administrative performance measures exceed mean for all VA medical centers (VAMC).
7. Meet all access to care standards.
8. Evidenced Based Health Care measures meet or exceed VA and DoD mean.
9. Satisfactory clinical and facility inspection outcomes from external oversight/accreditation groups, including but not limited to:
   a. Joint Commission
   b. VA Office of Inspector General (OIG)
   c. DoD OIG
   d. VA Office of the Medical Inspector
   e. Navy Bureau of Medicine and Surgery (BUMED) Medical Inspector General (MEDIG)
   f. American Association of Blood Banks
   g. United States Food and Drug Administration (FDA)
   h. VA OIG Combined Assessment Program (CAP) Reviews
   i. Occupational Safety and Health Administration.
10. Officer promotion/retention and enlisted advancement/retention meet or exceed Department of Navy (DON) means.
11. Information Management/Information Technology (IM/IT) implementation timeline met and no negative impact on patient safety.
12. Staff satisfaction and other appropriate measures identified VA and DoD as benchmarks.
13. Relative Value Unit (RVU)/Relative Weighted Product RVU/RWP/Dental Weighted Value production meets Business Plan targets.
14. Maintain pre FHCC academic and clinical research missions,
15. Trainee Satisfaction as measured by the Learner Perception Survey.

1

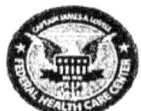

CAPTAIN JAMES A. LOVELL
FEDERAL HEALTH CARE CENTER
FISCAL YEAR 2013
BUDGET CALL
DEPARTMENT SUMMARY WORKSHEET

Directorate: Patient Care
Department: Dept of Amb Med Care
Division: Primary Care
Section: Internal Medicine

Amb Care Med All Other (60)
APPN: 0160
FCP: 2123

SAG/FSF (DOD): M8/YR

SPENDING HISTORY:	1st Qtr.	2nd Qtr.	3rd Qtr.	4th Qtr.	Total
FY10 (N/A)					
FY11 (EOY w/logistics)	$0	$74,443	$0	$0	$74,443
FY12 Plan (w/logistics):	$117,507	$3,360	$3,359	$3,359	$127,585

FY 2013 - FUNDING REQUESTED:

SUPPLIES:	1st Qtr.	2nd Qtr.	3rd Qtr.	4th Qtr.	Total
Logistics - FY12 (ref)	$3,360	$3,360	$3,359	$3,359	$13,438
Logistics - Office FY13	$0	$0	$0	$0	$0
Logistics - Medical FY13	$3,360	$3,360	$3,359	$3,359	$13,438
APPROVED	$0	$0	$0	$0	$0
Non Logistics - FY12 (ref)					$0
Non-Logistics Office - FY13	$0	$0	$0	$0	$0
Non-Logistics Medical - FY13	$0	$0	$0	$0	$0
APPROVED	$0	$0	$0	$0	$0

CONTRACTS:	1st Qtr.	2nd Qtr.	3rd Qtr.	4th Qtr.	Total
Contracts - FY12 (ref)	$114,147				$114,147
Contracts - FY13	$104,208	$0	$0	$0	$104,208
APPROVED	$0	$0	$0	$0	$0

FEE BASIS:	1st Qtr.	2nd Qtr.	3rd Qtr.	4th Qtr.	Total
Contracts - FY12 (ref)					$0
Contracts - FY13	$0	$0	$0	$0	$0
APPROVED	$0	$0	$0	$0	$0

	1st Qtr.	2nd Qtr.	3rd Qtr.	4th Qtr.	Total
FY 2013 - TOTAL REQUESTED:	$107,558	$3,360	$3,359	$3,359	$117,646

Is this amount more than FY12?   No
If YES, enclosure (4) MUST be completed.

	1st Qtr.	2nd Qtr.	3rd Qtr.	4th Qtr.	Total
FY 2013 - TOTAL APPROVED:	$0	$0	$0	$0	$0

Point of Contact for Budget Call issues:
(required field)

	First Name	Last Name	Rank	Phone Number
Department Head				
Budget Preparer				

WORKLOAD (DSS)	1st Qtr Oct-Dec	2nd Qtr Jan-Mar	3rd Qtr Apr-Jun	4th Qtr. Jul-Sep	Total	% Variance
FY10	0	0	0	0	0	
FY11	8694	8245	9951	11073	35963	
FY12	0	0	0	0	0	
					0	0.00%

encl (1)

Appendix IV: GAO Contact and Staff Acknowledgments

GAO Contact	Debra A. Draper, (202) 512-7114 or draperd@gao.gov
Staff Acknowledgments	In addition to the contact named above, Marcia A. Mann, Assistant Director; Jill K. Center; Regina Lohr; and Rasanjali Wickrema made key contributions to this report. Lisa A. Motley provided legal support, and Jennie F. Apter assisted in message and report development.

GAO's Mission	The Government Accountability Office, the audit, evaluation, and investigative arm of Congress, exists to support Congress in meeting its constitutional responsibilities and to help improve the performance and accountability of the federal government for the American people. GAO examines the use of public funds; evaluates federal programs and policies; and provides analyses, recommendations, and other assistance to help Congress make informed oversight, policy, and funding decisions. GAO's commitment to good government is reflected in its core values of accountability, integrity, and reliability.
Obtaining Copies of GAO Reports and Testimony	The fastest and easiest way to obtain copies of GAO documents at no cost is through GAO's website (www.gao.gov). Each weekday afternoon, GAO posts on its website newly released reports, testimony, and correspondence. To have GAO e-mail you a list of newly posted products, go to www.gao.gov and select "E-mail Updates."
Order by Phone	The price of each GAO publication reflects GAO's actual cost of production and distribution and depends on the number of pages in the publication and whether the publication is printed in color or black and white. Pricing and ordering information is posted on GAO's website, http://www.gao.gov/ordering.htm. Place orders by calling (202) 512-6000, toll free (866) 801-7077, or TDD (202) 512-2537. Orders may be paid for using American Express, Discover Card, MasterCard, Visa, check, or money order. Call for additional information.
Connect with GAO	Connect with GAO on Facebook, Flickr, Twitter, and YouTube. Subscribe to our RSS Feeds or E-mail Updates. Listen to our Podcasts. Visit GAO on the web at www.gao.gov.
To Report Fraud, Waste, and Abuse in Federal Programs	Contact: Website: www.gao.gov/fraudnet/fraudnet.htm E-mail: fraudnet@gao.gov Automated answering system: (800) 424-5454 or (202) 512-7470
Congressional Relations	Katherine Siggerud, Managing Director, siggerudk@gao.gov, (202) 512-4400, U.S. Government Accountability Office, 441 G Street NW, Room 7125, Washington, DC 20548
Public Affairs	Chuck Young, Managing Director, youngc1@gao.gov, (202) 512-4800 U.S. Government Accountability Office, 441 G Street NW, Room 7149 Washington, DC 20548